T0068104

PROGRESSIVE HEALTH CARE

Critical Health Care Information

Mary Duram, LMSW

authorHOUSE®

AuthorHouse™
1663 Liberty Drive
Bloomington, IN 47403
www.authorhouse.com
Phone: 1-800-839-8640

First published by AuthorHouse   01/21/2012

ISBN: 978-1-4685-4494-7 (sc)
ISBN: 978-1-4685-4493-0 (ebk)

Library of Congress Control Number: 2012901132

Printed in the United States of America

Contents

Acknowledgements

Special "thanks" to those individuals who gave freely of their time and talents to help ensure the accuracy, ease of use and design features of this booklet: Bruce Weaver, PA-C, President & CEO, AAging Better In-Home Care; Robert A. Ancker, M.D. Board Certified, American Board of Family Medicine, Board Certified Hospice and Palliative Medicine (CAQ), Medical Director, Hospice of North Idaho; Hunter Doherty "Patch" Adams, M.D. American physician, social activist, citizen diplomat and author. He is the founder of the Gesundheit Institute Arlington Virginia; Jonnie Bradley of CRServices, Publisher/Editor of *The Wise Guide* a bi-yearly senior resource magazine.

Mary Duram, LMSW, graduated from Eastern Washington University with a Masters of Social Work degree, specializing in Aging and Advocacy programs. Mary is the founder of Progressive Health Care as well as being a contract social worker. She chose her degree path after many years in the Assisted Living, Retirement, and Long Term Care fields, forming her philosophy: "To help individuals stay as independent as possible, at their highest level of functioning, for as long as possible." Mary helps her clients navigate the resource system to find the best possible programs for their individual needs.

Durable Power Of Attorney
And Emergency Information

The following Advanced Directives have been created:
(Check all that apply)

_____ Living Will

_____ Durable Power of Attorney for Health Care

_____ POST

Status _____ Full code

Status _____ Comfort Measures

Status _____ I am an organ donor

State Health Care Directive Registry Filing   Id_____ Password_____

See Page 25 for state web listings.

Please contact: _____ at _____
                          (Name)   (Address)

and _____ for more information.
        (Telephone)

I wish for the additional person(s) to be contacted in case of an emergency for emotional and family support.

Please contact   _____ at _____
                          (Name)   (Telephone)

Please contact   _____ at _____
                          (Name)   (Telephone)

Medical Diagnosis/Conditions

Blood Type_____

Continuum Of Care

Hospitalization

1. _____
   (Name of Facility)

   _____
   (Address)

   _____
   (City/State)   (Phone)

2. _____
   (Name of Facility)

   _____
   (Address)

   _____
   (City/State)   (Phone)

Assisted Living

_____
(Name of Facility)

_____
(Address)

_____
(City/State)   (Phone)

Long Term Care

_____
(Name of Facility)

_____
(Address)

_____
(City/State)   ·   (Phone)

Hospice Care

_____
(Name of Facility)

_____
(Address)

_____
(City/State)   (Phone)

NOTE: These listings are my preference but, I understand that due to medical circumstances, facility location, placement availability, or emergency situations, I will be taken where I can obtain immediate medical care.

Health Care Practitioners
And Specialists

This is a list of my personal health care team including:

Examples (Primary Care Physician, Cardiologist, Gastroenterology, Dermatology
Ophthalmology, Podiatry, Dentist/Denturist, Neurologist
Nutrition/Dietary, Ophthalmologist, Optometry)

Name _____ Discipline _____

_____
               (Address)   (City)

_____
               (Phone)   (Fax)

Name _____ Discipline _____

_____
               (Address)   (City)

_____
               (Phone)   (Fax)

Name _____ Discipline _____

_____
               (Address)   (City)

_____
               (Phone)   (Fax)

Name _____ Discipline _____

_____
(Address)   (City)

_____
(Phone)   (Fax)

Name _____ Discipline _____

_____
(Address)   (City)

_____
(Phone)   (Fax)

Name _____ Discipline _____

_____
(Address)   (City)

_____
(Phone)   (Fax)

Name _____ Discipline _____

_____
(Address)   (City)

_____
(Phone)   (Fax)

Current Medication List

This page lists the medications I currently take as of (date) _____. Updates will be added to maintain accurate records.

Medication   Dose   Frequency

_____
_____
_____
_____
_____
_____
_____
_____

Vitamins Or Supplements

Supplement   Dose   Frequency

_____
_____
_____
_____
_____
_____
_____
_____

Medication And Supplement Updates

Update _____
    (Day/Month/Year)

Medication   Dose   Frequency

_____
_____
_____
_____
_____
_____
_____
_____

Medication And Supplement Updates

Update _____
    (Day/Month/Year)

Medication/Supplement   Dose   Frequency

_____
_____
_____
_____
_____
_____
_____
_____

Medication And Supplement Updates

Update _____
        (Day/Month/Year)

Medication   Dose   Frequency
_____
_____
_____
_____
_____
_____
_____
_____

Medication And Supplement Updates

Update _____
        (Day/Month/Year)

Medication/Supplement   Dose   Frequency

_____
_____
_____
_____
_____
_____
_____
_____

Medication And Supplement Updates

Update _____
        (Day/Month/Year)

Medication/Supplement   Dose   Frequency

_____

_____

_____

_____

_____

_____

_____

_____

Medication Allergies/Sensitivities
And Reactions

Medication Allergies   Reactions

_____
_____
_____
_____
_____
_____
_____
_____

Food Allergies   Reactions

_____
_____
_____
_____
_____
_____
_____

Allergies   Reactions
Examples (Bee stings, grass, mold,
Latex, soap, cologne, etc.)

_____
_____
_____
_____
_____
_____
_____

Insurance And/Or Supplements

Company _____ _____
                                                        (Telephone Number)
Address_____

Policy Number_____ Group Number_____

Email Address _____

Other information _____

Company _____ _____
                                                        (Telephone Number)
Address_____

Policy Number_____ Group Number_____

Email Address _____

Other information _____

Company _____ _____
                                                        (Telephone Number)
Address_____

Policy Number_____ Group Number_____

Email Address _____

Other information _____

Company _____ _____

(Telephone Number)

Address_____

Policy Number_____ Group Number_____

Email Address _____

Other information _____

Company _____ _____

(Telephone Number)

Address_____

Policy Number_____ Group Number_____

Email Address _____

Other information _____

The Event Of My Death

Funeral Arrangements

Please contact _____ Phone_____
He/She will be arranging my burial along with the mortuary and cemetery personnel. Thank you.

_____ I wish to be buried

_____ I wish to be cremated

Funeral Home Or Crematorium

Funeral Home _____ Phone: _____

Address _____

City/State _____

Cemetery _____ Phone _____

Address _____

City/State_____

Plot Number/Location _____

What Is An Advanced Directive?

An Advanced Directive is a document that helps an individual to protect their right to refuse or limit medical treatment(s) in the event that they lose the ability to make decisions for themselves. It is suggested that an individual speaks with their physician or other health care providers about their medical condition when completing their directives. Individuals may also want to consider any personal, cultural or spiritual beliefs which could effect their health care decisions. To assure individual rights the advanced directive is composed of two sections:

Living Will And The Durable Power Of Attorney For Health Care.

Note: These documents are legally binding only if the person completing them is a competent adult (at lease 18 years of age) or is an emancipated minor.

Legalizing your document is state specific. Many states require that your documents are witnessed and notarized while; other states require an individual only sign their Living Will and Durable Power of Attorney for Health Care. However, if you think there is a possibility that your document may be disputed at any time, you may consider having your signature witnessed and/or notarized.

The Living Will

This document lets an individual state their medical care wishes in the event that they are terminally ill or in a persistent vegetative state and can no longer make medical decisions for themselves. The living will becomes effective when two doctors certify that an individual is terminally ill and death will occur with or without the use of life-sustaining treatments or that they are in a persistent vegetative state.

The Durable Power Of Attorney For Health Care (DPOAH)

This section of the document allows an individual to appoint someone to make decisions about their medical care, including decisions about life support, if they are no longer able to speak for themselves. It is important to note that the Durable Power of Attorney for Health Care appoints someone to speak for an individual any time they are unable to make their own medical decisions, not only at the end of life. The person appointed may be referred to as the health care agent, attorney-in-fact or proxy. An individual may choose a second or third agent to step in if the first person named as agent is unable, unwilling or unavailable to act for you.

Within the Durable Power of Attorney (state specific) is a section entitled **"Statement of Desires, Special Provisions, and Limitations"**. In this section an individual may add personal instructions pertaining to their health care. However, by doing so an individual might unintentionally restrict their agent's power to act in their best interest. One of the main reasons for naming an agent is to have someone who can respond flexibly to any unforeseen situations that may arise. It is suggested that instead of adding specific instruction; that an individual speaks with their health care agent to discuss what they feel would be an acceptable "quality of life". Your agent must make decisions that are consistent with your known desires.

Who Can Be Appointed As An Agent?

The person named can be a family member or someone trusted to make serious decisions. That person should clearly understand the individual's wishes and be willing to accept responsibility for making medical decisions.

Important Facts Individuals Should Know.

In the event of an emergency the Living Will and Durable Power of Attorney for Health Care may not be effective. Ambulance personnel are required to provide cardiopulmonary resuscitation (CPR) unless they are given a separate order which states otherwise. These orders are designed for people whose poor health gives them little chance of benefiting from CPR. The orders must be signed by a physician, and ambulance personnel must be instructed not to attempt CPR if an individual's heart or breathing should stop. *These orders are called a "POST/ POLST" order and can be obtained from your physician*

A pregnant patient's Living Will may not be honored due to restriction in state law.

Who Cannot Be Named As An Agent/Proxy?

Each state has set its own requirements for who can or cannot be named as an individual's agent or proxy. Some states such as Montana have no restriction and your agent/proxy can be a family member, health care worker, or physician.

Other states such as Idaho and Washington State will not allow:

- The individual's doctor or treating health care provider.
- Any employee of an individuals treating health care provider, unless he or she is related to you.
- Operators of a community care facility; or employee of a community care facility, unless he or she is related to you.

The advanced directive for your individual state will clarify who can or cannot be named.

What Should Be Done With The Documents After Completing Them?

Keep the original signed document is a secure but accessible place. This document should not be placed in safe deposit boxes or any other security box that would keep others from having access to them.

Photocopies of the original should be made and given to your agent, alternative agents, doctor(s), clergy or anyone else you wish to be involved in your health care. If an individual enters a nursing home or hospital, photocopies of the document should be placed in the medical file.

Individuals should talk often with their agent and alternative agents, doctor(s), clergy and family and friends about their wishes concerning medical treatment. It is important to have these discussions if/when an individual's medical condition.

If an individual wishes to make changes to their documents after they have been signed and witnessed, a new document must be completed.

Changing The Durable Power Of Attorney For Health Care

A Durable Power of Attorney for Health Care can be revoked at any time regardless of an individual's mental condition.

Steps to revoke include: canceling, defacing, obliterating or other wise destroying the document or directing another to do so in your presence.

An individual can sign a written revocation; or orally express their intent to revoke the document.

Note: an individual can always revoke their Living Will and Durable Power of Attorney for Health Care

POST Or POLST

Depending on the state in which you live an individual can complete a Physicians order of Sustained Treatment (POST) or a Physicians order for Life Sustaining Treatment (POLST). The POST/POLST form helps patients clearly express their health care wishes and transforms those wishes into medical orders. Because the form stays with the individual it is durable across the entire health care setting; it is effective at home, in skilled nursing facilities, hospitals and during emergency medical transport. Because the POST/POLST form is a medical order it must be discussed with and signed by your physician and may be obtained in his or her office. Having a POST/POLST helps insure an individual's medical treatment wishes are followed but, does not completely replace advanced directives. Having a Durable Power of Attorney naming an agent for surrogate decision making is a very helpful addition.

Health Insurance Priority Acquisition Act (HIPAA)

Privacy Rule

The HIPAA Privacy Rule regulates the use and disclosure of Protected Health Information (PHI) held by "covered entities" (generally, health care clearinghouses, employer sponsored health plans, health insurers, and medical service providers that engage in certain transactions.) PHI is any information held by a covered entity which concerns health status, provision of health care, or payment for health care that can be linked to an individual. Covered entities must disclose PHI to the individual within 30 days upon request. They also must disclose PHI when required to do so by law, such as reporting suspected child abuse to state child welfare agencies.

A covered entity may disclose PHI to facilitate treatment, payment, or health care operations, or if the covered entity has obtained authorization from the individual. However, when a covered entity discloses any PHI, it must make a reasonable effort to disclose only the minimum necessary information required to achieve its purpose.

The Privacy Rule gives individuals the right to request that a covered entity correct any inaccurate PHI. It also requires covered entities to take reasonable steps to ensure the confidentiality of communications with individuals. Covered entities must also keep track of disclosures of PHI and document privacy policies and procedures. The Privacy Rule requires covered entities to notify individuals of uses of their PHI.

The State Registry

Individuals may choose to register their POST/POLST, Advanced Directives and Living Will with their home state. The registry can be found through the Secretary of State web site with complete instructions and forms needed. Although having the paper copies of your documents is necessary they are not forms individuals carry with them in all situations. Depending on your state you may be sent a card or other form of identification to carry with you that will instruct you on how to access your information on the registry. Most importantly the registry is accessible by medical personnel during emergency and non-emergent medical treatment; and is the quickest and most direct way for health care providers to access your health care and medical treatment wishes.

Advanced Directive Web Sites

Many web sites are available with state specific "free" Advanced Directive forms and registration. Your local advanced directives can be found by typing (your state name) and advanced directives in the interned address bar. The following list is a small sampling of web sites that offer advanced directive forms for all 50 states. This author does not endorse any one web address.

www.LegacyWriter.com
www.AdvancedDirectives.Rocketlawyer.com
www.OnlineForms.LawDepot.com
www.uslfw.com/formslist.shtm
www.caringinfo.org

Individuals who receive medical treatment in a bordering state are encouraged to complete an advanced directive and/or POST/POLST for each state. Advanced directives may be written specifically and applicable only for that state. This will ensure that your health care wishes are known and can be carried out.

State Registration
Of Advanced Directives

To register your advanced directives with your state, visit the state Attorney General's Office web site.

Organ Donation

According the Wikipedia web site, www.wikipedia.org: Under the law of the United States, the regulation of organ donation is left to states within the limitations of the Uniform Determination of Death Act, the National Organ Transplant Act, and the United Network for Organ Sharing (UNOS). Each state's Uniform Anatomical Gift Act seeks to streamline the process and standardize the rules among the various states. Many states have sought to encourage the donations to be made by allowing the consent to be noted on the driver's license. Donor registries allow for a central information center for an individual's wish to be a donor. Some individuals may wish to make an anatomical gift by donating their organs or body to a teaching hospital or medical university.

Additional Notes Or Information

Additional Notes Or Information

Additional Notes Or Information

Additional Notes Or Information

Additional Notes Or Information

Additional Notes Or Information

Additional Notes Or Information

Additional Notes Or Information